Homemade Perfume
20 Best Organic Perfume Recipes That Will Make You Smell Great

Table of content

Introduction

Smelling nice is such an essential part of life. We all want to smell good and wearing perfume is one of the best ways we do that. As women, we wear perfume if not every day, at leas on special occasions. We want to smell nice for the opposite sex, for co-workers, for friends and most importantly for ourselves.

However, we've started to learn about all the terrible things that are found in perfume sold in stores and marketed to women around the world. Perfume can be linked to all sorts of health problems in both men and women, but for decades we didn't know about it.

Now that more and more women know about the risks associated with wearing perfume, they are asking questions and want to know about alternatives. They want to wear something that will still have them smelling nice, but not expose them to the chemicals that put their bodies and health at risk.

The great thing is that organic perfume is the perfect alternative. The other problem is that most women don't have the time, patience or money to spend on making organic perfume. That's okay. Organic perfume doesn't have to take loads of time preparing, nor does it need to cost an exuberant amount of money.

After reading through this article, you'll understand the basics of making your own perfume and have twenty recipes to get you started.

Chapter 1 – Why You Should Make the Switch to Organic

So let's take a minute to talk about the dangers of using regular perfumes from the store. Many people experience different health concerns that are connected to perfumes. Although research can't directly connect the two, many scientists believe they are connected.

Because fragrance companies don't want to release their recipes, so others can't copy them. Because of this, they don't have to list their ingredients on the label of their products, and thus can basically put anything inside. Analysts have recently found troubling things inside perfumes that are linked to things like sperm damage, breast milk, headaches, other epidemiological problems, etc.

Ultimately the fact that they don't have to list their ingredients on their labels is a huge loophole in the system and troubling to most people. When buying a fragrance, most people don't think about the ingredients, but instead just think about the smell. They trust companies won't put things in their products that would damage or hurt their consumers. And if not putting trust in the company, a consumer puts trust in the government to regulate something like this.

Unfortunately that regulation doesn't exist for something like this. The Food and Drug Administration doesn't assess the safety of spray on products. They are stretched too thin to work on fragrances and instead focus their efforts elsewhere. This is disturbing information for those people who have trusted their bodies to companies for years with certain fragrances they believed were safe.

Unfortunately, these fragrances are full of chemicals that aren't safe and were never safe for the body. The potential health risks associated with using store-bought perfumes are through the roof and getting higher with every study. Companies are taking advantage of customers and consumers who fail to recognize that they are use shortcuts and failings in the government to their advantage. And who are the ones to pay for it? The average citizens. People like you and me who just don't know any different.

But the fact is now you do know different. Now you are going to know and be armed with the truth and you are going to be able to do something different. And the best part about it is that the alternative we're going to suggest for you is simple, easy to accomplish and affordable. Oh, and the best part – it smells amazing!

We will give you the tools and recipes to create some great perfumes to have for every time of year. You won't regret switching over. The other option you'll have is to create your own perfume that is completely unique to you. We'll teach you the basics of making a perfume and then you can customize it with essential oils to make it the perfect scent.

Let's get started talking about making and creating all the perfect types of organic perfumes you can make.

Chapter 2 – Different Essential Oil Combinations for Organic Perfumes

There are so many wonderful different combinations of essential oils out there that it's hard to know where to get started sometimes. We'll talk about how to build your base, but then the possibilities are endless. You'll have to get some of your favorite essential oils start mixing and matching them together in order to build your own favorites. Then you will have a unique scent that is all your own.

However in the mean time, we can also give you a few recipes that are some of our favorites to get you started. These recipes will give you something to build your own scents. That way you will have some of the best essential oils, too. Then as you have the essential oils to work with, you can find those that you really like and start to build a library of scents.

DIY Perfume in Non-Spray Bottle

Ingredients

4 T 100 Proof Vodka

2 T Jojoba Oil, Olive Oil, Almond Oil

1 T Distilled Water

30-60 drops of Essential Oil

Directions

Add all ingredients into a dark glass jar and place in a dark, cool place to let sit for four to six weeks. This particular recipe is generic with essential oils, but shows you the building block for which many of the recipes below will build off of. If you want to experiment with creating your own perfume, here is where to start. Create this base, and then start adding essential oils to find your own unique scent that you love.

The four to six week waiting period will give the oils time to blend with the vodka, oil and water. After six weeks, your perfume is ready to use. You can either keep the perfume in the same jar you prepared it in or transfer it into a pretty perfume bottle.

Note: 100 proof vodka can be very difficult to find in a liquor store, so if you can't find 100 proof, you can settle for 80 proof and your perfume will turn out just fine. Just remember the higher the proof the better.

DIY Perfume for Spray Bottle

Ingredients

4 T 100 Proof Vodka

2 T Distilled Water

30-60 drops of Essential Oil

Directions

Add all ingredients into a dark glass jar and place in a dark, cool place to let sit for four to six weeks. This particular recipe is generic with essential oils, but shows you the building block for which many of the recipes below will build off of. If you want to experiment with creating your own perfume, here is where to start. Create this base, and then start adding essential oils to find your own unique scent that you love.

The four to six week waiting period will give the oils time to blend with the vodka and water. After six weeks, your perfume is ready to use. You can either keep the perfume in the same jar you prepared it in or transfer it into a pretty perfume bottle.

You will notice the major difference between the first two recipes is the fact that the first has a carrier oil (jojoba, almond or olive oil and the second does not. The first perfume is just a little thicker and won't work in a spray bottle. So any recipe you see in this section that contains a carrier oil can't be used in a spray perfume bottle. However, if you want to modify the recipe and use the oil combination without the carrier oil, that's easily done!

Note: 100 proof vodka can be very difficult to find in a liquor store, so if you can't find 100 proof, you can settle for 80 proof and your perfume will turn out just fine. Just remember the higher the proof the better.

Jasmine Perfume

Ingredients

4 T 100 Proof Vodka

2 T Distilled Water

Jasmine Blend of Essential Oils

    40 drops Jasmine Oil

    10 drops Vanilla Extract

    10 drops Lavender Oil

Directions

In a glass bottle or jar, mix all the essential oils and the vodka. Leave the mixture for two days. After two days, add the distilled water and shake gently. Place the mixture in a dark and cool place and leave for three to four weeks. After four weeks, move the perfume from the glass bottle into a spray bottle. Your perfume is ready for use!

Note: 100 proof vodka can be very difficult to find in a liquor store, so if you can't find 100 proof, you can settle for 80 proof and your perfume will turn out just fine. Just remember the higher the proof the better.

Light Perfume

Ingredients

2 T 100 Proof Vodka

1 T Distilled Water

10 drops Tangerine Oil

10 drops Grapefruit Oil

10 drops Rosemary Oil

Directions

Add all ingredients into a dark glass jar and place in a dark, cool place to let sit for four to six weeks. (Note: Rosemary is a little stronger than the other two oils. You may want to add a little of this at a time and smell the mixture to decide how much of this you really want to add before adding all ten drops.)

This will give the oils time to blend with the vodka and water. After six weeks, your perfume is ready to use. You can either keep the perfume in the same jar you prepared it in or transfer it into a pretty perfume bottle (spray or otherwise).

Note: 100 proof vodka can be very difficult to find in a liquor store, so if you can't find 100 proof, you can settle for 80 proof and your perfume will turn out just fine. Just remember the higher the proof the better.

Refresh Perfume

Ingredients

4 T 100 Proof Vodka

2 T Jojoba Oil

1 T Distilled Water

20 drops Tea Tree Oil

20 drops Lavender Oil

20 drops Spearmint Oil

Directions

Add all ingredients into a glass jar. The spearmint oil is a little strong, so you may want to add it last and a little at a time until you reach your desired scent. After all ingredients are combined in the jar, place it in a dark and cool location to sit for four to six weeks.

After six weeks your perfume is ready to use. You can leave it in the jar or transfer it to another glass container while using it.

Note: 100 proof vodka can be very difficult to find in a liquor store, so if you can't find 100 proof, you can settle for 80 proof and your perfume will turn out just fine. Just remember the higher the proof the better.

Citrus Perfume

Ingredients and Supplies

Glass Container with Lid (for making and blending)

Fun Glass Perfume Bottle (for storage and use)

2 T jojoba oil

4 T 100 proof vodka

60 drops of essential oils

      Sweet Orange

      Grapefruit

      Peppermint

      Lavender

      Chamomile

2 T distilled water

Directions

Add the jojoba oil and the alcohol to the glass container and mix until they are well combined. After the oil and the alcohol are combined, it's time to add the oils. It's important that you add the oils in the correct order. Add them like this —

      15-20 drops of grapefruit

      15-20 drops of sweet orange and then 5-10 drops of peppermint

      5 drops of lavender and 5 drops of chamomile

Finally the last step is to add the distilled water. If you can and have the ability, add the distilled water by using a dropper (like a medicine dropper for little kids).

Place a lid on top. Find a dark and cool place to store the perfume for up to six weeks. The longer you store the perfume the better the scent will blend.

After six weeks, transfer the perfume to your nice bottle and enjoy!

Note: 100 proof vodka can be very difficult to find in a liquor store, so if you can't find 100 proof, you can settle for 80 proof and your perfume will turn out just fine. Just remember the higher the proof the better.

Fresh Scent Perfume

Ingredients

4 T 100 Proof Vodka

2 T Jojoba Oil

1 T Distilled Water

30 drops grapefruit oil

20 drops ginger oil

15 drops vetiver oil

Directions

Add all ingredients into a dark glass jar and place in a dark, cool place to let sit for four to six weeks.

The four to six week waiting period will give the oils time to blend with the vodka, oil and water. After six weeks, your perfume is ready to use. You can either keep the perfume in the same jar you prepared it in or transfer it into a pretty perfume bottle.

Note: 100 proof vodka can be very difficult to find in a liquor store, so if you can't find 100 proof, you can settle for 80 proof and your perfume will turn out just fine. Just remember the higher the proof the better.

Girls Night Out Perfume

Ingredients

4 T 100 Proof Vodka

2 T Jojoba Oil

1 T Distilled Water

40 drops rose oil

20 drops lime oil

20 drops vetiver oil

Directions

Add all ingredients into a dark glass jar and place in a dark, cool place to let sit for four to six weeks.

The four to six week waiting period will give the oils time to blend with the vodka, oil and water. After six weeks, your perfume is ready to use. You can either keep the perfume in the same jar you prepared it in or transfer it into a pretty perfume bottle.

Note: 100 proof vodka can be very difficult to find in a liquor store, so if you can't find 100 proof, you can settle for 80 proof and your perfume will turn out just fine. Just remember the higher the proof the better.

First Date Perfume

Ingredients

4 T 100 Proof Vodka

2 T Jojoba Oil

1 T Distilled Water

30 drops sweet orange oil

20 drops ylang-ylang oil

10 drops cedarwood oil

Directions

Add all ingredients into a dark glass jar and place in a dark, cool place to let sit for four to six weeks.

The four to six week waiting period will give the oils time to blend with the vodka, oil and water. After six weeks, your perfume is ready to use. You can either keep the perfume in the same jar you prepared it in or transfer it into a pretty perfume bottle.

Note: 100 proof vodka can be very difficult to find in a liquor store, so if you can't find 100 proof, you can settle for 80 proof and your perfume will turn out just fine. Just remember the higher the proof the better.

Mountain Retreat Perfume

Ingredients

1 T Olive Oil

8 drops spruce oil

4 drops fir needle oil

4 drops cedarwood oil

2 drops vetiver oil

2 drops bergamot oil

Directions

Add all the essential oils to a small glass bottle and roll between your hands to mix together. Then add the carrier oil and do the same to mix together. Smell the combination and decide if additional essential oils are needed. You can use this kind of perfume immediately.

Smells Like Summer Perfume

Ingredients

1 T Almond Oil

20 drops lavender oil

10 drops chamomile oil

8 drops cardamom oil

2 drops cedarwood oil

2 drops rose oil

Directions

Add all the essential oils to a small glass bottle and roll between your hands to mix together. Then add the carrier oil and do the same to mix together. Smell the combination and decide if additional essential oils are needed. You can use this kind of perfume immediately.

Chapter 3 – How to Make Organic Solid Perfumes

Making a solid perfume is perfect to have in the bathroom, but also in your purse for when you're out and about and need a little freshening up. The idea of having a solid perfume is so wonderful; you'll regret that you haven't had them around forever. Here is the basic idea of how to put one together and then some recipes to get you started creating your own.

DIY Solid Perfume

Ingredients

3 T beeswax beads (sold online or at most craft stores)

3 T olive oil

40 drops of essential oils (give or take)

Storage container(s)

Directions

Using a double boiler, melt the beeswax beads until fully melted. (You can also substitute them for beeswax shavings, but the beads are extremely convenient if you can find them.) Remove the melted beeswax from the heat and immediately stir in the olive oil until the mixture is smooth.

Add in your favorite combination of essential oils. The scent will be a little strong while the mixture is hot, but will fade slightly when it cools, so keep that in mind as you mix. Before it cools, pour the mixture into your storage container(s).

Let the perfume set for a day or at least overnight. Use a finger or two to rub the perfume on the inside of your wrists and you'll smell fabulous all day long. The perfume will last 12 months.

Travel Solid Perfume

Ingredients and Supplies

Lots of Small Containers (lip balm type containers, bead cases, etc. – you can find them online and order bulk if you want, or try craft stores)

35-40 drops Honeysuckle Oil

1 T Beeswax (grated)

1 ½ T Almond Oil

Directions

In a double boiler, add the beeswax and let it melt until it is completely melted. Then add your almond oil to the beeswax and stir until the two are completely combined. Then slowly add your essential oil to the mix. A craft stick works really well to mix everything together. Then pour your mixture into the containers you've chosen.

These work well as gifts or to take in your purse, gym bag, etc. They don't melt except at extremely high temperatures (beware of leaving one in your car during the summer), but you're probably safe just about everywhere else. You can even trust giving them to older children. They won't spill when opened and older girls love the idea of wearing perfume.

Lavender Solid Perfume

Ingredients

2 T grated beeswax

2 T almond oil

10 drops of lavender oil

Small container

Directions

Melt the beeswax in a double boiler on the stove until it is thoroughly melted. Once it is melted, add the almond oil and mix the two together. Finally stir the lavender oil into the mixture until everything is well mixed. Then pour the mixture into a small container to let it set.

Lavender isn't a particularly strong scent. It mixes well with vanilla, mint, rose or sweet orange. This is a great solid perfume to experiment with adding other oils and scents if you want to mix and match until you find a combination that suits you.

Lavender is a very soothing scent. So you can use it to help you fall asleep. It can also help with headaches and jet lag.

Sandalwood Solid Perfume

Ingredients

4 T beeswax (already grated)

4 T almond oil

30 drops sandalwood oil

30 drops vanilla extract

25 drops grapefruit oil

20 drops bergamot oil

Container(s) This recipe makes about 1/3 cup of solid perfume so pick containers accordingly

Directions

First heat the beeswax in a double boiler until it is completely melted. Use low heat so it doesn't burn. After it is melted stir in the almond oil and take it off the heat. Mix them together so they are completed mixed. Next start to add the essential oils, one at a time, stirring each in individually. Do this quickly so the mixture doesn't start to harden. After all the oils are added, pour the mixture into whatever containers you've chosen to store your perfume in and let it harden.

You can start using your perfume immediately after it hardens (usually within six hours) and will last up to nine months. If you would like it to last longer, switch the almond oil with jojoba oil (24 months) or olive oil (12 months).

The "Double L" Solid Perfume

Ingredients

2 T Almond Oil

1 T beeswax (grated)

20 drops lavender oil

10 drops rosemary oil

5 drops lemongrass

Directions

Use your double boiler and melt your beeswax on your lowest heat setting to keep it from burning. After it is done melting, add the almond oil and stir until they are well combined. Remove the mixture from the heat and let it cool down for a half a minute, but not too long. Then add all the essential oils in the order listed in the recipe. Quickly pour the mixture into the container(s) you plan to store the perfume in for use. Let them cool and then they are ready for immediate use.

Chapter 4 – Other Perfume Options

Sometimes you are just looking for something that's a little different. It doesn't mean that you don't love the idea of a solid perfume or the traditional spray bottle, but something a little different is just nice once in a while. When you're looking for something different, there are a few options to consider that might be nice to have around.

These options might take a little longer to make or might require extra supplies, but you can always take these into consideration when deciding whether or not to make them and adding them to your cabinet of perfumes.

Roll-On With Essential Oils

Ingredients and Supplies

Roll-on Vials (can be purchased online)

Almond Oil (enough to fill your roll-on vials)

15-20 drops of your favorite essential oil or a combination

Directions

First fill the roll-on vial with almond oil almost to the top, but leave just a little room for your essential oil. Then add your combination of essential oil(s) to the top and swirl or shake after putting the top back on. Voila! You have a roll-on perfume that is most convenient!

Body Powder

Ingredients and/or supplies

2 C Organic Cornstarch

1 cotton ball

Favorite essential oil (or combination) in a spray bottle

Large Mason Jar with lid (or equivalent)

Directions

Take all supplies/ingredients into the bathroom or next to the kitchen sink. Take your cotton ball and the essential oil spray and give the cotton ball a really good spray. (You can also use a perfume that you've made with essential oils if you have one in a spray bottle.) Don't soak it so it's dripping, but spray the cotton ball probably 30 times. So you don't feel like you're wasting perfume, you can hold the cotton ball inside the Mason jar so the residue from the spray goes on the inside of the jar.

Then drop the cotton ball in the bottom of the Mason jar. Add the cornstarch on top of the cotton ball, but make sure you leave at least two inches (or about a quarter of the jar) empty at the top. Give the jar a good shake (probably for about a minute). Put the jar in a dark place and remember to shake it for the next three days two times a day.

After three days, your body powder is ready for use. You can fish out the cotton ball if it is easily accessible, but it's not necessary. When you come across it, just toss it in the garbage, but don't worry about it until you do. The best time to apply body powder is right after you've showered or bathed and your pores are open. Enjoy!

Clove Lotion and Perfume Bar

Ingredients

4 T Almond Oil

4-5 T Beeswax

4-8 drops Jasmine Oil

4 drops Clove Oil

4 drops vanilla extract

Storage Container(s)

Directions

First pour the almond oil into a small container and add each of the essential oils slowly. It is difficult to add just the allotted number of drops, but try to keep them as close as possible or the scent will end up overwhelming. Stir everything together.

Use a double boiler to heat the beeswax until it's completely melted. Then add the oil mixture to the melted beeswax and stir to combine. After everything is mixed together quickly transfer to your storage containers and let them harden.

If you want to speed up the process, you can put them in the freezer. Otherwise let them harden overnight. To use, just apply a small amount with one or two fingers.

The difference between a lotion bar and solid perfume is the amount of beeswax you add to the mixture. The more beeswax you add it becomes less like a solid perfume and more like a lotion bar. When your perfume is done cooling, it just might slide out of the container if you turn in upside down. Now you have a lotion bar that you can rub on (kind of like deodorant), but in places where you would normally use lotion like your hands or feet.

You can keep it in the storage container(s) when you aren't using it, but use it as a lotion bar otherwise. It's up to you how much beeswax you want to add to see how solid it becomes.

Body Spray

Ingredients

½ C Jojoba Oil

1 t vanilla extract

4 drops clove oil

Medium glass spray bottle

Directions

Combine all the ingredients into the medium spray bottle and shake well to combine. You may want to add the clove a drop at a time smelling in between. Open and smell or give a small spray to see how well everything has combined. You can add more vanilla if needed. The clove may be a little overpowering, so adding more vanilla will help to balance it out. Add it a ¼ t at a time in between each drop of clove if necessary.

Chapter 5 – A Word on Essential Oils

We won't dwell long on this topic, but since essential oil are such a huge part of making your own perfume there are few really important things to understand about essential oils if you aren't familiar with them or haven't really dealt with them in the past. So let's spend just a little bit of time talking about essential oils.

1) **Cheaper isn't Better** – You can purchase essential oils just about any-where these days. The unfortunate part is that you really will get what you pay for when it comes to essential oils. You will learn the hard way that if you don't pay just a little bit more for good quality essential oils, you'll be dumping in a lot more to get a good scent out of your perfume. So when we talk about adding just 10-20 drops of something, you'll end up drop-ping in half your bottle to get the same results.

2) **Where Can You Buy Them?** – There are local distributors selling good quality essential oils everywhere, but you can also purchase them online if you can't find a distributor in your area. You don't have to buy a certain brand or from a certain distributor, just higher quality in order to get the same kind of results you really want.

3) **Oil Blending** – Oil blending isn't perfect and it's not a science either. The recipes in this book weren't discovered the first time people sat down to try and make their own perfumes. Like most creative things, they were

made through trial and error and mostly through having fun. Oil blending shouldn't be stressful, but should be a fun, new adventure.

Start by going somewhere that has essential oils (it can even be a place that sells low-quality ones), and smell them. Find your favorites or narrow out some of the scents you don't like. This will give you an idea about where you'd like to start. Then blend two or three oils together and see how they blend. Some oils blend well together – like citrus oils.

Take notes while you blend, because maybe you'll come across an oil blend you really like, but if you haven't been taking notes, you won't remember what you blended or how many drops you put in of which oils. You'll want to recreate your perfume for future uses and you'll only be able to do that if you've been taking notes.

Conclusion

Making your own perfume is a wonderful new step and journey that will allow you to tap into your creative side while also saving your health by no longer using store bought perfume. It's time to clean out your bathroom and rid yourself of body sprays, perfumes and any other scent related things you might have lurking around the house.

You are now educated and armed with the knowledge of how to make your own perfume, and you know that it's really not that difficult. Rather you decide to completely make your own scent by trying out oil blending or take one of these already created recipes, you can have a perfume ready to go by this afternoon or tomorrow.

It's time to take the responsibility of your health and your body into your own hands and do something fun at the same time by making your own perfume! Grab a friend and make some together. You'll not only be doing them a favor, but you can have a good time, too!

FREE Bonus Reminder

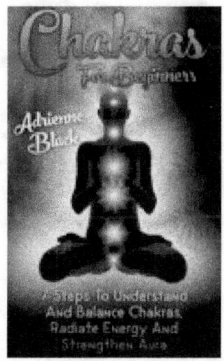

If you have not grabbed it yet, please go ahead and download your special bonus E book *"Chakras for Beginners. 7 Steps To Understand And Balance Chakras, Radiate Energy, And Strengthen Aura"*.

Simply Click the Button Below

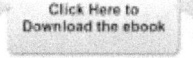

OR Go to This Page

http://lifehacksworld.com/free

BONUS #2: More Free & Discounted Books & Products

Do you want to receive more Free/Discounted Books or Products?

We have a mailing list where we send out our new Books or Products when they go free or with a discount on Amazon. Click on the link below to sign up for Free & Discount Book & Product Promotions.

=> **Sign Up for Free & Discount Book & Product Promotions** <=

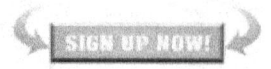

OR Go to this URL

http://zbit.ly/1WBb1Ek